CARDIAC DIET FOR HEART HEALTH

A Comprehensive Guide to the Nourish, Protect, and Thrive with the Essential Cardiac Diet Strategies

Petersen Kohler

TABLE OF CONTENTS

CHAPTER ONE

Introduction

The Significance of Heart Health:

Living a long and happy life depends on keeping your heart healthy. The good news is that many risk factors for heart disease can be controlled with dietary and lifestyle changes. Heart disease is nevertheless one of the major causes of death worldwide. The purpose of this book is to give you useful information and recommendations on a cardiac diet for heart health so that you may make the best decisions and safeguard your heart.

Who This Book Is For:

People who have been diagnosed with or are at risk of heart disease, as well as those who wish to take proactive measures towards improved heart health, should read this book. This guide will give you the information and resources you need to make wise dietary decisions, whether you're a worried person trying to lower your risk of heart problems or someone who has to manage their heart condition.

How to Use This Book: To get the most out of this book, familiarize yourself with the principles of eating a heart-healthy diet. We'll look at the food selections, portion sizes, and nutritional components that can support heart health. It's critical to keep in mind that, although eating is very important, a healthy lifestyle that includes regular exercise and stress reduction should also be followed. This guide will assist you in creating a balanced diet for your heart that meets your specific needs by providing helpful hints, meal plans, and recipes.

Make informed decisions to support your heart health journey by using it as a resource for meal planning, grocery shopping, and decision-making.

Knowing About Heart Health

It is crucial to have a thorough grasp of heart health before creating a cardiac diet that will promote heart health. The heart is an amazing organ that is essential to preserving our general health. Understanding the structure and operation of the heart, identifying prevalent heart health problems, and identifying the risk factors connected with heart disease are the first steps towards developing a heart-healthy diet plan.

The Heart's Anatomy And Function:

Slightly to the left of the center, in the chest, lies the muscular organ that houses the human heart. Its size is comparable to that of a closed fist, and its function is to circulate oxygenated blood throughout the body. There are two atria (upper chambers) and two ventricles (bottom chambers) in the heart.

The left side of the heart pumps oxygen-rich blood from the lungs to the rest of the body, while the right side pumps deoxygenated blood from the body to the lungs for oxygenation. Electrical impulses that govern the contraction of the cardiac muscles and preserve a constant blood flow are responsible for the heartbeat.

Typical Heart Health Problems:

The following cardiac health conditions can have a serious negative effect on a person's well-being:

1. The artery that supplies blood to the heart becomes clogged with plaque when a person has Coronary Artery Disease (CAD). Heart attacks, angina, and other cardiovascular problems might result from it.

2. Heart Failure: The inability of the heart to pump blood efficiently results in heart failure, which manifests as weariness, fluid retention, and dyspnea.

3. Heart rhythm irregularities, or arrhythmias, can result in palpitations, lightheadedness, or fainting.

4. Heart valve damage or abnormalities cause ventricular heart disease, which impairs blood flow.

5. Congenital Heart Defects: A few people are born with structural heart defects that may need to be treated medically.

Potential Hazards For Heart Disease:

Creating a cardiac diet for heart health requires an understanding of the risk factors for heart disease. Numerous risk factors can be altered to lower the risk of heart disease, while others, like genetics, are unchangeable:

1. Poor Diet: Heart disease can be exacerbated by a diet heavy in cholesterol, sodium, Trans and saturated fats, and added sugars.

2.   Physical Inactivity: Not getting enough exercise on a regular basis raises the risk of heart disease.

3. Smoking: Because smoking destroys blood arteries and lowers blood oxygen levels, it is one of the main risk factors for heart disease.

4.   Hypertension, or high blood pressure: High blood pressure raises the risk of heart disease and puts strain on the heart.

5.   Elevated Cholesterol: An accumulation of plaque in the arteries may result from elevated levels of LDL (low-density lipoprotein) cholesterol.

6. Obesity: Carrying excess weight raises your risk of heart disease.

7.   Diabetes: Individuals with diabetes, especially if their blood sugar levels are not

well controlled, are more likely to develop heart disease.

We can better customize a cardiac diet that promotes heart health and lowers the risk of cardiovascular disease by understanding the complexities of heart health, including the structure and function of the heart, common heart health disorders, and modifiable risk factors. We will go into more detail on creating a meal plan that is heart-healthy and lifestyle modifications that can support heart health in the next sections.

Basics Of Cardiac Diets

1. The Diet's Role In Heart Health:

An essential part of maintaining heart health is following a cardiac diet. Our diets have a direct effect on our risk of heart disease.

Conditions including excessive blood pressure, high cholesterol, and atherosclerosis can be prevented and managed with the support of a heart-healthy diet.

2. Micronutrients And Macronutrients: The proper ratio of carbs, proteins, and fats is the main emphasis of a cardiac diet that is balanced. It's critical to increase unsaturated fats and decrease trans and saturated fats. Additionally, heart health is greatly influenced by micronutrients such as vitamins, minerals, and antioxidants—especially potassium, magnesium, and other minerals.

3. Heart Health And The Mediterranean Diet: The Mediterranean diet is frequently advised in order to promote heart health. Lean proteins, nuts, fruits, veggies, whole grains, and olive oil are all highlighted. It is high in fiber, antioxidants, and monounsaturated fats, all of which are beneficial to cardiovascular health.

4. Advice For A Heart-Healthy Diet: Take into account the following advice in order to keep your diet heart-healthy:

• Eat less sodium to lower blood pressure.

• Eat less processed and high-sugar foods.

• For a range of nutrients, including a selection of vibrant fruits and vegetables.

• Opt for whole grains rather than refined ones.

• Choose lean protein sources such as fish, chicken, and plant-based foods.

• Employ nutritious cooking techniques like baking, steaming, and grilling.

Observe serving sizes to control your caloric intake.

• Limit sugar-filled beverages and stay hydrated with water.

• Track and control cholesterol levels by consuming less trans and saturated fat.

By incorporating these principles into your diet on a daily basis, you can lower your risk of heart-related problems and greatly improve heart health. For individualized nutritional advice and guidance, always seek the advice of a licensed dietitian or healthcare expert.

CHAPTER TWO

Selecting Heart-Healthy Foods For A Cardiac Diet

Sustaining a heart-healthy diet lowers the risk of cardiovascular disease and improves general health. Proper meal selection can significantly contribute to heart health promotion. When it comes to foods that are good for your heart, keep the following points in mind:

1. Fruits And Vegetables: Fruits and vegetables are a great source of fiber, antioxidants, and other nutrients. These meals offer protection against heart disease, lower blood pressure, and lower cholesterol. Make an effort to eat a range of colorful foods, such as citrus fruits, cruciferous vegetables, berries, and leafy greens.

2. Whole Grains: Rich in fiber and offering a consistent supply of energy, whole grains include brown rice, oats, and whole wheat. They can lower the risk of heart disease and help control blood sugar levels. For your bread, pasta, and cereals, choose whole-grain alternatives rather than processed grains.

3. Lean Proteins: For a diet that promotes heart health, lean protein sources including fish, chicken, lentils, and tofu are great options. They can aid in maintaining a healthy weight, which is essential for heart health, and have less saturated fat. Include omega-3 fatty acids, which are particularly healthy for the heart, in your diet by eating fatty seafood like salmon.

4. Good Fats: Not every fat has negative effects. Foods high in nuts, seeds, avocados, and olive oil include monounsaturated and polyunsaturated fats, which can lower bad cholesterol and lower the risk of heart disease. Reduce your intake of trans fats, which are frequently present in processed and fried meals, as well as saturated fats from dairy and red meat.

5. Herbs And Spices: A few herbs and spices have the ability to prevent heart disease in addition to adding taste to your food. For instance, the anti-inflammatory qualities of garlic, turmeric, and ginger can help improve heart health. Add these to your food to enhance its flavor and nutritional value.

6. Foods To Avoid: Restricting or avoiding particular foods is essential for maintaining a diet that is heart-healthy. These consist of:

• Highly Processed Foods: Processed foods can contain excessive levels of sodium, added sugars, and harmful fats. They may be a factor in obesity and hypertension.

• Sugary Drinks: Consuming sugary drinks, such as soda and fruit juices with added sugar, is linked to weight gain and a higher risk of heart disease. Choose unsweetened alternatives, herbal tea, or water instead.

• Excessive Sodium: Eating a diet heavy in sodium raises the risk of heart disease and can cause hypertension. Consider how much salt you consume and, where possible, opt for lower-sodium foods.

• Excess Alcohol: Drinking too much alcohol can damage the heart and other organs, even while moderate alcohol use may have some heart-healthy benefits. If you decide to drink, make sure it's moderate.

You may dramatically lower your risk of heart disease and encourage a better, happier life by concentrating on these heart-healthy dietary choices and avoiding those that could compromise your cardiovascular health. To design a customized nutrition plan that meets your unique needs and health objectives, speak with a medical practitioner or a registered dietitian.

Meal Preparation And Portion Management

1. Meal Planning: It's critical to plan meals that are well-balanced and comprise a range of nutrient-rich foods when implementing a cardiac diet. Make sure to include whole grains, an abundance of fruits and vegetables, lean proteins (fish, poultry, and plant-based sources), and whole grains. This keeps salt and saturated fats in check while ensuring you get the nutrients you need.

2. Portion Control: Maintaining heart health requires regulating portion sizes. Overconsumption of even healthful meals can have negative effects. Make use of visual cues. For example, divide your plate into parts for each food type or compare your serving of meat to a deck of cards. Reduced serving sizes can aid in controlling caloric intake and avert overindulgence.

3. Meal Timing: You can balance blood sugar levels and reduce overeating by eating at regular intervals and avoiding large stretches of time between meals. Smaller, more frequent meals and snacks are advised throughout the day to sustain energy levels and avoid severe hunger, which can result in bad eating choices.

4. Eating Out Wisely: Maintaining a cardiac diet when dining out can be difficult. Make healthier selections by looking up restaurant menus online in advance, choosing grilled or steamed dishes over fried ones, and asking for dressings and sauces on the side to manage portion sizes.

By incorporating these ideas into your diet, you can lower your risk of cardiovascular issues and better manage your heart health. Always get advice from a qualified nutritionist or healthcare provider to develop a customized food plan that suits your individual requirements and tastes.

Preparing Heart-Healthy Dinners

Sustaining a cardiac diet is crucial for heart health in order to lower the risk of cardiovascular illnesses and improve general health. Making heart-healthy meals is one of the diet's main tenets. While preparing heart-healthy meals, keep the following basic ideas in mind:

1. Cooking Techniques: Select cooking techniques that call for little to no additional fat while preparing heart-healthy meals. These methods are great: baking, grilling, broiling, steaming, and poaching. These techniques lessen the demand for bad fats while preserving the flavors of food. Steer clear of deep-frying, as this may add an excessive quantity of trans and saturated fats to your diet.

2. Tasting Without Adding Too Much Salt: Heart health depends on consuming less salt, or sodium. To add flavor to your food, think about utilizing herbs, spices, and other seasonings in place of too much salt. Spices like cumin, paprika, and garlic, together with herbs like basil, thyme, and rosemary, can improve the flavor of your food without adding additional salt. For extra taste, lemon juice, vinegar, and citrus zest are also excellent substitutes.

3. Recipe Adaptations: It's a proactive move to make your favorite foods heart-healthy. Replace high-cholesterol and high-saturated-fat items with less unhealthy options. For example, use olive oil in place of butter, whole grains in place of refined grains, and lean meat or plant-based protein sources. Other positive adjustments are to use less sugar and more veggies in your cooking.

4. Sample Recipes For Heart Health:

Here are a few heart-healthy recipe examples to get you started with the cardiac diet:

Salmon on the grill with a lemon-dill sauce:

• Components:

• Four fillets of salmon

- Two tsp of olive oil

- Two tsp freshly squeezed lemon juice

- One tsp. dried dill

- Add pepper and salt to taste.

- Directions:

Set the grill's temperature to medium-high.

Combine the olive oil, lemon juice, dill, salt, and pepper in a small bowl.

Apply the olive oil mixture to the salmon fillets.

The salmon should flake easily with a fork after grilling it for 4–5 minutes on each side.

Accompany with quinoa and cooked asparagus on the side.

Mediterranean Salad with Chickpeas:

Components:

• Two cups of rinsed and drained canned chickpeas

• One cup of chopped cucumber

• One cup of tomato dice

• Chopped red onion, half a cup

• 1/4 cup of freshly chopped parsley

• Three tsp olive oil

• Half a tablespoon of lime juice

• One teaspoon of oregano, dried

• Add pepper and salt to taste.

Guidelines:

Chickpeas, cucumber, tomato, red onion, and parsley should all be combined in a big bowl.

Mix the olive oil, lemon juice, oregano, salt, and pepper in another bowl.

Drizzle the salad with the dressing and toss to coat.

Before serving as a cool side dish, place in the refrigerator for a minimum of half an hour.

You may enjoy tasty, heart-healthy dishes that promote your cardiovascular health by preparing your meals using these cooking methods, flavoring strategies, and recipe adjustments. Keep in mind that maintaining long-term heart health requires consistency in your food choices.

CHAPTER THREE

Adjustments To Lifestyle For Heart Health

1. Exercise And Physical Activity: A heart-healthy diet must include both regular exercise and physical activity. Walking, swimming, and cycling are examples of aerobic exercises that can help control weight, lower blood pressure, and enhance cardiovascular fitness. Aim for 150 minutes or more per week of moderate-to-intense activity or 75 minutes or more of vigorous exercise.

2. Stress Management: Prolonged stress has a detrimental effect on cardiac health. Include stress-reduction methods in your everyday routine, such as yoga, meditation, or deep breathing. By lowering the risk of heart disease, these measures can help lessen the release of stress hormones.

3. Quitting Smoking: One of the main risk factors for heart disease is smoking. To overcome your addiction to nicotine, get help from medical specialists, prescription drugs, or support groups.

4. Alcohol Use: Excessive alcohol use can be harmful, although moderate alcohol consumption may offer some heart-protective benefits. Limit your alcohol intake to moderate amounts for heart health, which are usually one drink for women and two for men each day.

5. Heart Health And Sleep: Getting enough sleep is essential for heart health. Aim for seven to nine hours of good sleep every night. Heart disease risk is increased by factors like obesity and hypertension, which are exacerbated by poor sleep quality and insufficient sleep. To support improved heart health, establish a regular sleep routine and create a comfortable sleeping environment.

Drugs And Cardiovascular Health

Heart Condition Medications

Medications are essential for treating a variety of cardiac problems and preserving heart health. Healthcare providers frequently recommend these drugs to assist in regulating and enhancing heart function. The particular ailment, its severity, and the unique characteristics of the patient all influence the prescription selection. The following list of common heart disorders includes the drugs that are used to treat them:

1. Hypertension, or high blood pressure: Heart disease is significantly increased by high blood pressure. ACE inhibitors, beta-blockers, diuretics, and calcium channel blockers are among the medications that are commonly used to lower blood pressure and lessen cardiac strain.

2. Coronary Artery Disease (CAD): Drugs such as statins are used to reduce cholesterol and stop plaque from accumulating in the arteries. Aspirin and other antiplatelet medications help avoid blood clots that can result in heart attacks.

3. Heart Failure: Drugs such as beta-blockers, diuretics, ACE inhibitors, and angiotensin receptor blockers (ARBs) benefit patients with heart failure by managing fluid retention, enhancing the heart's pumping capacity, and easing symptoms.

4. Arrhythmias: Anti-arrhythmic medications may be used to treat irregular heartbeats. Warfarin and other blood-thinning drugs are sometimes used to stop blood clots.

Medication Administration:

Heart medication needs to be managed properly to maximize benefits and reduce dangers. Here are some important things to think about:

1. Frequent Consultations: In order to evaluate the effectiveness of drugs and alter dosages as needed, patients should schedule routine check-ups with their healthcare provider.

2. Comprehending Medication: It's critical that patients comprehend the goals of each

drug, any possible adverse effects, and how it affects their heart health.

3. Observe dosing Instructions: It's important to stick to the recommended dosing schedule. Modifying drug intake or missing doses can have a negative impact on heart health.

4. Polypharmacy Management: Individuals who have various heart diseases could take several drugs. It's critical to maintain an up-to-date record of all medicines, notify medical professionals of any new ones, and be mindful of any possible interactions.

Possible Adverse Reactions:

The adverse effects of heart medication can differ from one medication to the next. Frequent adverse effects may include changes in blood pressure, headaches, exhaustion, nausea, or dizziness. Serious or even fatal adverse effects can occur occasionally. Patients should notify their healthcare practitioner of any unexpected symptoms as soon as possible.

The Value Of Following Medication Instructions:

A key element of treating cardiac diseases and preserving heart health is medication adherence, or taking drugs as directed by a doctor. This is the reason it's crucial:

1. Effectiveness: Good adherence guarantees that drugs function as prescribed, which aids in the efficient treatment and management of cardiac disorders.

2. Complications can be prevented by taking medication as prescribed. These complications

include heart attacks, strokes, and increasing heart failure.

3. Better Quality of Life: People with heart diseases may get symptom relief, increased capacity for activity, and an all-around higher quality of life if they take their prescribed drugs as directed.

4. Decreased Hospitalizations: Adhering to medication regimens helps lessen the number of hospital stays for heart-related problems.

Healthcare professionals can collaborate with patients to address issues, streamline treatment regimens, and offer educational materials in order to improve medication adherence. Involving caregivers or family members can also assist in guaranteeing that patients follow their prescription schedules.

In summary, medicine plays a critical role in the management of heart health. For those with heart-related problems, controlling cardiac disorders, lowering risks, and improving general well-being depend on proper knowledge, management, and adherence to recommended drugs. For individualized advice and direction on heart drugs, always seek the opinion of a healthcare expert.

Observation And Proactive Steps

1. Frequent Health Check-Ups: Keeping an eye on your heart health requires routine health check-ups. They make it possible for medical professionals to evaluate your general health and pinpoint any possible danger factors. These examinations can aid in the early detection of heart-related problems and allow for prompt intervention.

2. Blood Pressure And Cholesterol Monitoring: Two of the biggest risk factors for heart disease are high blood pressure and elevated cholesterol. It is essential to regularly check your cholesterol and blood pressure readings. If necessary, prescription drugs and lifestyle modifications may be suggested to maintain these figures within a healthy range.

3. Diabetes Management: Heart issues and diabetes are frequently related. Controlling your blood sugar levels is essential for heart health if you have diabetes.

Following a cardiac diet can assist with blood sugar regulation and lower the chance of diabetic heart problems.

4. Weight Management: Heart health depends on maintaining a healthy weight. Being overweight raises the risk of heart disease and puts strain on the heart. Maintaining a healthy weight or losing extra weight requires frequent exercise in addition to adhering to a good diet.

5. Heart-Healthy Lifestyle Choices: Developing heart-healthy lifestyle choices is a long-term preventive strategy. Eating a diet high in fruits, vegetables, whole grains, lean meats, and low-fat dairy products while reducing your intake of trans and saturated fats is one of these behaviors. Maintaining heart health also requires controlling stress, avoiding drinking, and smoking, and engaging in regular physical activity.

By implementing these preventative and monitoring practices into your daily routine, you can lower your risk of heart disease and improve your heart health in general. It's crucial to speak with a healthcare expert to develop a customized strategy that best fits your unique requirements and situation.

Summary

How To Get And Keep Your Heart Healthy:

To sum up, a cardiac diet is an essential part of keeping your heart healthy. Although heart disease is still the world's greatest cause of death, heart-healthy eating can greatly lower the chance of developing cardiovascular problems.

We have discussed the need to cut back on salt, minimize saturated and trans fats, up fiber intake, and include heart-healthy foods like fruits, vegetables, whole grains, and lean proteins in our diets. These food options can help control weight, and lower blood pressure, and cholesterol—all of which improve heart health.

But it's crucial to keep in mind that eating a heart-healthy diet is only one aspect of the picture. The maintenance of a healthy weight, regular exercise, and stress reduction are also essential for overall cardiovascular well-being. Furthermore, before making any big nutritional changes, especially if you have underlying medical concerns, it's imperative to speak with a healthcare provider.

The Path Ahead:

Achieving and sustaining heart health is a lifelong journey. It's about making a commitment to long-term lifestyle improvements rather than quick cures. Although it could occasionally seem difficult, the benefits are definitely worth the work. These are important things to remember when you set out on this journey:

1. Making heart-healthy decisions a regular part of your life requires consistency. These modest adjustments will add up to major heart health gains over time.

2. Seek assistance: Don't be afraid to get in touch with dietitians, medical specialists, and support groups. They can offer direction, inspiration, and useful advice catered to your particular needs.

3. Stress should be considered since it might have a detrimental effect on heart health.

Include stress-relieving practices in your regimen, such as yoga, meditation, or deep breathing exercises.

4. Frequent check-ups: To keep an eye on your heart health, make an appointment with your doctor on a frequent basis. They can assist you in monitoring your development and modifying your plan as necessary.

5. Keep yourself informed: Keep learning about heart-healthy decisions and recent advancements in the area. Acquiring knowledge is an effective means of improving your cardiac health.

Supplementary Materials And Assistance:

It can be difficult to maintain a diet and lifestyle that are heart-healthy, but you're not alone in this attempt. You have access to a wealth of tools and sources of assistance to guide you along the way:

1. Healthcare professionals: For individualized advice and support catered to your unique requirements and medical conditions, speak with your physician or a certified dietitian.

2. Support groups: You can connect with people who have similar objectives and life experiences by joining a support group or an online community. It's a fantastic method to get advice and support from those traveling similar paths.

3. Educational resources: There is a plethora of information available on diets, fitness regimens, and heart-healthy meals in books, websites, and apps. To keep things interesting and fresh, keep up with current events and try out new meals and workout routines.

4. Mobile apps: You can track your nutrition, exercise, and general health progress with a variety of apps available. They can be very useful resources for maintaining motivation and focus.

5. Heart-healthy organizations: To assist you in maintaining a heart-healthy lifestyle, organizations such as the American Heart Association and the World Heart Federation offer a wealth of information, publications, and tools. Additionally, these groups frequently organize campaigns and events to increase public awareness of heart health issues.

You can dramatically lower your risk of heart disease and live a longer, healthier life by adopting a heart-healthy diet, changing your lifestyle sustainably, and asking professionals and like-minded people for support.

THE END

www.ingramcontent.com/pod-product-compliance
Lightning Source LLC
Chambersburg PA
CBHW060814260726
48660CB00002B/940